VITAMINS

The Missing Link in Your Health

Dr. David D. Reid

TABLE OF CONTENT

"YOU CAN'T CONTROL EVERYTHING IN YOUR LIFE BUT, YOU CAN CONTROL WHAT YOU PUT IN YOUR BODY"

INTRODUCTION TO VITAMINS

What are Vitamins, Why Do We Need Them, and How Do They Function in the Body?

Vitamins are chemical substances that are vital for sustaining healthy health. They serve a key part in several biological activities such as development, metabolism, and the immune system. Vitamins are required in modest quantities, but they are necessary and cannot be manufactured by the body in significant amounts. Hence, they must be acquired from food or supplementation.

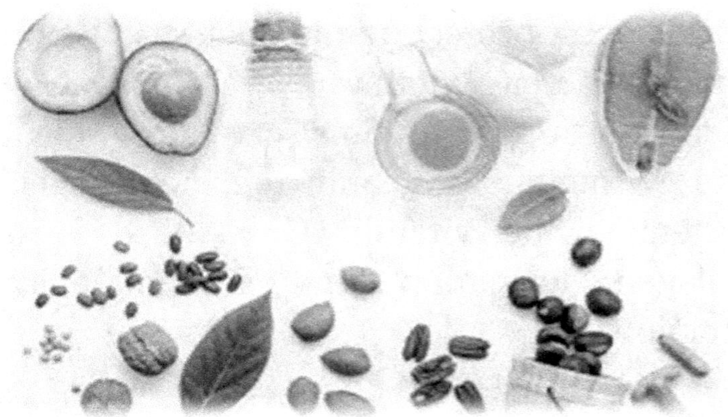

There are two basic kinds of vitamins: fat-soluble and water-soluble. Fat-soluble vitamins (vitamins A, D, E, and K) dissolve in fats and oils and are stored in the body's fatty tissues. Water-soluble vitamins (vitamins B and C) dissolve in water and are not stored in the body to a substantial level. Instead, they are eliminated via urine, thus they need to be supplied periodically.

Each vitamin has a special purpose in supporting healthy health. For example, vitamin A is vital for eyesight and immunological function, while vitamin D is needed for bone health and calcium absorption. Vitamin E functions as an antioxidant, protecting the body's cells from harm, whereas vitamin K is involved in blood clotting. B vitamins serve a key role in energy metabolism and the neurological system, while vitamin C is needed for collagen formation and immunological function.

Vitamins may be derived from a number of sources. Certain vitamins are present in a broad variety of meals, whereas others are highly concentrated in particular foods. For example, vitamin C is plentiful in citrus fruits, strawberries, and broccoli, while vitamin A is rich in liver, sweet potatoes, and carrots. Vitamin D may be gained from exposure to sunshine, as well as through fortified dairy products and fatty fish.

Deficiencies in vitamins may lead to numerous health concerns. For example, vitamin A deficiency may induce night blindness, while vitamin D deficiency can lead to rickets. Vitamin C deficiency may result in scurvy, a condition marked by weakness, anemia, and gum disease. On the other hand, excessive ingestion of some vitamins may be damaging to health, such as vitamin A toxicity, which can cause liver damage.

Vitamins are vital elements that are needed in little quantities to sustain optimum health. They are categorized into two categories: fat-soluble and water-soluble vitamins. Each vitamin has a distinct job in the body, and shortages or excesses may contribute to numerous health concerns. It is vital to have a balanced and varied diet to guarantee appropriate consumption of vitamins and to contact a healthcare practitioner before taking supplements.

CHAPTER 1: HEALTH BENEFITS OF VITAMINS

With today's hurried and modern lifestyle, it may be tricky to acquire enough of the nutrients necessary for the body from the food you eat. Generally, the body requires a fixed quantity of minerals and vitamins to function. Every person has a recommended daily amount (RDA) of all essential vitamins. For instance, the body requires vitamin K for the blood to coagulate and vitamin D to absorb calcium. Some nutrients may also help support biological functions, like the skin's integrity and collagen.

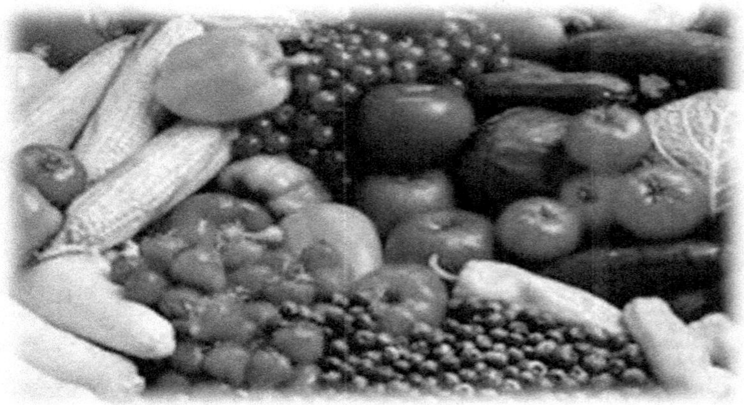

Yet, one of the things to keep in mind when taking vitamins is that they're not a replacement for a healthy diet nor for antibiotics and other treatments, but they're merely a supplement to the food you consume. For instance, if you have genital herpes, you should still be taking the needed meds and complementing it with a suitable supplement, like Luminance RED. This is because a solid diet together with taking the essential vitamins and supplements often is needed to successfully manage herpes.

These are some of the various benefits of taking vitamins:

Promotes Healthy Aging

As much as you aspire to stay young forever, nobody is exempt from aging. Additionally, the older you grow, the more you'll need to care for your physical health. Regrettably, as you age, it is tougher for the body to absorb the much-needed nutrients and particular medicines may deplete nutrients further.

An excellent and straightforward strategy to look after your health is by consuming vitamins. As you get older and begin to confront inadequacies, there are various vitamins that may aid reset your nutritional level.

Reduces Anxiety and Stress

The minerals and vitamins in your daily multivitamins may greatly lessen levels of anxiety and stress. To turn food into energy, the body utilizes B vitamins. Such vitamins are also important to preserve your neurological system running effectively. Consuming vitamins consistently may replenish your body's supply of such vitamins.

Boosts Your Cardiovascular Health

Some vitamins, such as magnesium, CoQ10, and B vitamins, all aid promote a healthy cardiovascular system. Consequently, if you're one of the people who worry about cardiovascular health in general, eating vitamins may help retain your heart healthy. So be careful to combine it with eating heart-healthy foods.

Covers Your Nutritional Bases

Everyone does their best to eat appropriately, yet certain nutrients could be difficult to gain through food alone. Whenever you take vitamins regularly, you may be certain that you'll complete your daily wants for all the important minerals and vitamins.

Supports Your Immune System

With today's current milieu, your immune system is more crucial than ever, so it only makes sense that you seek to nurture it as much as possible.

If you're thinking of the traditional vitamins related to enhancing your immune system, it's vitamin C, which is renowned for being a potent antioxidant. Moreover, you may also take vitamins E and D to strengthen your immunity.

You may receive vitamins by purchasing them from a local pharmacy or a vitamin shop. Sadly, reliance on these vitamins isn't enough. You still need to eat appropriate fruits and green leafy vegetables.

Keeps Body in Good Working Order

One of the key benefits of taking vitamins regularly is that it maintains the body in optimum operational condition. Essentially, vitamins work hard to maintain the body running properly and aid drive the vital actions that are required daily.

Every nutrient you acquire from vitamins is on a mission to deliver benefits that assist you to accomplish your health goals in no time.

Improves Your Eyesight

Taking particular vitamins has been reported to support your eye wellness. Vitamins E, C, A, and selenium are good for strengthening eyesight. Moreover, ingesting a combination of zeaxanthin, lutein, and vitamins may lessen the risk of macular degeneration.

The time spent looking at the screens on Televisions, laptops, and phones has grown over the years, which is one of the key reasons why most people have impaired eyesight. For example, if you've been working in front of your computer for 8 hours a day, your eyes will most surely suffer.

An efficient technique to counteract vision decline is taking measures and employing vitamins often. Eating meals finest for your eyesight or eye health is also a superb tip, especially if you aren't used to taking vitamins consistently or tend to forget to take one sometimes.

Keeps Your Bones Strong

You certainly know that calcium is required for healthy bones. Nevertheless, did you know that vitamin D is essential for calcium to complete its job?

The skin also creates vitamin D upon direct solar exposure, however, the use of sunscreen, poor skin absorption, and weak winter sunlight may work against the development of this vital nutrient. Even if vitamin D is added to milk, most folks don't eat dairy products regularly.

Increases Brain Function

Another benefit of consuming vitamins is that they may help increase brain function. It may also encourage greater mental health as other conditions like depression and anxiety may be due to vitamin deficits. Thus, there's no harm in taking vitamins that may assist combat such deficits. Just assure you consume excellent vitamins solely. If you don't sure which vitamins to take are best for you, ask your doctor for help.

Improves Healthy Metabolism

B vitamins, such as riboflavin, thiamin, B6, B12, biotin, and folate interact with particular enzymes in your body to absorb energy from fats, carbohydrates, and protein. Consuming a good diet and remaining physically active also assist maintain a healthy metabolism, which are vital elements for your general health and healthy aging.

Promotes Healthy Skin and Hair

One of the benefits of ingesting vitamins is that it encourages healthier hair and skin. If you're battling with your skin, whether it's eczema, dry skin, or acne, there are special vitamins out there, mainly vitamins E, A, and C that assist minimize such issues.

If you're battling with split ends or thinning hair, vitamins B3 and C are the greatest selections to grow fuller.

CHAPTER 2: THE RISK OF VITAMINS DEFICIENCY

You may assume nutritional inadequacies are a thing of the past, encountered exclusively by sailors on lengthy sea journeys. Yet even today, it's possible to lack some of the key nutrients your body needs to operate efficiently.

Nutrient shortages impact biological functions and processes at the most fundamental cellular level. These activities include water balance, enzyme activity, neuron signaling, digestion, and metabolism. Addressing these inadequacies is critical for proper growth, development, and function.

Nutritional deficits may also lead to illnesses. For example, calcium and vitamin D shortages may induce osteopenia or osteoporosis, two disorders characterized by brittle bones and insufficient iron may induce anemia, which zaps your energy.

Telltale signs are frequently the first signal that you are short in one or more key vitamins or minerals. Here's how to spot seven common nutritional deficits.

Iodine plays a part in your metabolisms' general operation, protein production, and conversion to useable physiological compounds.

Calcium: Numb, Tingling Fingers and Irregular Heart Rhythm

Calcium is vital for keeping healthy bones and managing muscle and nerve function. Symptoms of significantly low calcium include numb, tingling fingers and irregular heart rhythms says the Cleveland Clinic. That said, there are no short-term, visible indications of calcium shortage.

Most individuals require 1,000 milligrams (mg) of calcium per day, however, women over 50 and men over 70 need 1,200 mg. You'll likely get enough from at least three cups of milk or yogurt a day. Cheese is another good source of calcium, but if you're not big on dairy, you can find this nutrient in calcium-fortified orange juice or breakfast cereal (check the nutrition facts label of the food to see if calcium has been added), and dark leafy greens like kale and broccoli, according to the NIH.

Vitamin D: Fatigue, Bone Pain, Mood Shifts, and More

This vitamin is another that's vital for bone health and may help prevent certain malignancies, according to the Cleveland Clinic. Signs of a vitamin D shortage might be nonspecific weariness, bone discomfort, mood changes, and muscular pains or weakness may develop in.

If it continues on long enough, a vitamin D deficit might lead to the weakening of the bones. The long-lasting deficit also may be connected with malignancies and autoimmune illnesses.

Most individuals require 15 micrograms (mcg) of vitamin D per day, while those older than 70 need 20 mcg. Patton advocates consuming three glasses of fortified milk or yogurt daily and eating fatty fish, such as salmon or tuna, twice a week, since these are foods that contain vitamin D; spending some time outdoors in the sunlight every day, too, as this is a fantastic source of the mineral. Fifteen to 30 minutes a few times a week of direct sunshine exposure should help.

Potassium: Muscle Weakness, Constipation, Irregular Heart Rhythm, and More

Potassium helps your heart, nerves, and muscles perform correctly and also supplies nutrition to cells while eliminating waste. Moreover, it's a helpful vitamin that helps balance sodium's detrimental influence on your blood pressure: It's vital in keeping a good blood pressure.

You might get low in potassium in the short term because of diarrhea or vomiting; excessive sweating; antibiotics, laxatives, or diuretics; excessive alcohol intake; or because of a chronic ailment such as renal disease. Signs of a deficiency include muscular weakness, twitches, or cramps; constipation; tingling and numbness; and an irregular heartbeat or palpitations.

For natural potassium supplies, try bananas, milk, acorn squash, lentils, kidney beans, and other legumes. Mature males require 3,400 mg per day, while women need 2,600 mg.

Iron: Fatigue, Shortness of Breath, Cold Hands and Feet, Brittle Nails, and More

Iron is vital to generate red blood cells, which transport oxygen throughout the body, according to the University of California in San Francisco. When iron levels go too low, there may be a deficit in red blood cells, resulting in a disease called anemia. Other populations at heightened risk of iron deficiency include menstruation women, developing persons (such as youngsters and pregnant women), and those following a vegan or vegetarian diet.

Anemia may leave you with symptoms like weakness and exhaustion, shortness of breath, a rapid pulse, pale complexion, headache, chilly hands and feet, a painful or swollen tongue, brittle nails, and desires for weird things like dirt. The symptoms may be so faint at first that you don't detect something's wrong, but as iron supplies grow more depleted, they will become more acute.

To raise iron levels, Patton advises consuming iron-fortified cereal, meat, oysters, beans (particularly lima, navy, and kidney beans), lentils, and spinach. Adult men and women over 50 require 8 mg per day, while adult women younger than 50 need 18 mg per day.

Vitamin B12: Numbness, Fatigue, Swollen Tongue, and More

Vitamin B12 supports the synthesis of red blood cells and DNA, and also enhances neurotransmitter function. Vegetarians and vegans may be at particular risk for vitamin B12 deficiency because plants don't make the nutrient, and people who've had weight loss surgery may also lack B12 because the procedure makes it difficult for the body to extract the nutrient from food.

Signs of severe B12 deficiency include tingling in the legs, hands, or feet; trouble with walking and balance; anemia; exhaustion; weakness; a swollen, inflamed tongue; memory loss and difficulty thinking. These symptoms might come on fast or gradually, and because there's such a broad variety of symptoms, you may not notice them for a time.

People require 2.4 mcg of B12 each day. It is most typically found in animal products, and Patton suggests fish, chicken, milk, and yogurt enhance your B12 levels. If you're vegan or vegetarian, I advise opting for items fortified with B12, such as plant-based milk and morning cereals. You can also get B12 in most multivitamins, but if you're in danger of being deficient, you may take a supplement, particularly containing B12.

Folate: Fatigue, Diarrhea, Smooth Tongue, and More

Folate, or folic acid, is a B vitamin that's especially crucial for women of reproductive age, which is why prenatal vitamins normally include a heavy dosage. Folate promotes healthy development and function and may lower the chance of birth abnormalities, especially those affecting the neural tube (the brain and spine). Folate shortage may lower the total number of cells and big red blood cells and induce neural tube problems in an unborn kid.

Signs of a folate shortage include weariness, irritability, diarrhea, poor development, and a smooth, tender-feeling tongue.

Women who potentially get pregnant should make sure they obtain 400 mcg of folic acid daily in addition to ingesting meals containing folate. Curiously, folate is best absorbed by the body in supplement form, with 85 percent absorbed from supplements and 50 percent from meals.

To receive folate from the diet, look for fortified cereals, beans, peanuts, sunflower seeds, whole grains, eggs, and dark leafy greens.

Magnesium: Loss of Appetite, Nausea, Fatigue, and More

Magnesium helps promote bone health and supports energy generation, and individuals require between 310 and 420 mg, depending on sex and age. While deficiency is rather rare in otherwise healthy persons, some drugs (including certain antibiotics and diuretics) and health disorders (such as type 2 diabetes and Crohn's disease) might decrease the absorption of magnesium or accelerate the loss of this vitamin from the body.

Magnesium shortage may induce a lack of appetite, nausea and vomiting, exhaustion, and weakness. In more severe situations, it may also lead to numbness and tingling, muscular cramps or contractions, seizures, abnormal heart rhythms, personality changes, or coronary spasms.

To help your levels return to normal, consume more magnesium-rich foods, such as almonds, cashews, peanuts, spinach, black beans, and edamame.

CHAPTER 3: THE TRUTH ABOUT VITAMINS SUPPLEMENT

When it comes to supplements, there's so much buzz about their potential advantages that it may be hard to discern reality from fantasy. Although it's true that vitamins and minerals are vital to health, it's not true that taking them in pill, capsule, or powder form particularly in mega doses is required or without dangers.

For one reason, nutritional supplements may occasionally interact with one other, as well as with over-the-counter (OTC) and prescription drugs. In addition, unlike medicines, the U.S. Food & Drug Administration (FDA) is not permitted to assess dietary supplements for safety and efficacy before they are sold. It's up to producers to guarantee that their goods do not include contaminants or impurities, is correctly labeled, and contain what they advertise. In other words, the regulation of dietary supplements is significantly less severe than it is for prescription or OTC pharmaceuticals.

But, according to the FDA, more than half of Americans use herbal or dietary supplements every day, with research by Grandview Research indicating the dietary supplements industry was valued at $151.9 billion globally in 2021.

Taken appropriately, certain supplements may benefit your health, while others may be useless or even hazardous. For example, a systematic analysis examining the possible effects of nutritional supplements on cardiovascular health, primarily heart attack and stroke, reveals that few supplements help prevent heart disease – only omega-3 fatty acids and folic acid were useful. The same went for dietary adjustments, except for a low-salt diet.

A study including self-reported dietary habits from a group of Americans connected daily doses of more than 1,000 milligrams (mg) of calcium to a higher risk of dying from cancer.

Additionally, the data indicated that persons who took in enough levels of magnesium, zinc, and vitamins A and K had a decreased risk of dying – but only if they acquired those nutrients from food rather than supplements.

Buyer beware. Many supplements on the market have not been carefully evaluated. Very few supplements have demonstrated to be of help. Many carry unsubstantiated health claims.

Confused? National Institutes of Health (NIH) fact sheets may give thorough information on the advantages and hazards of various vitamins and minerals, as well as herbal supplements. And if you're treating an underlying health issue (particularly if you're on medication) or are pregnant or nursing, play it safe and have a talk with your healthcare team before adding any new supplement to your routine.

Although supplement fads come and go, these are seven supplements that historically have been popular and in all instances, experts advocate using them cautiously, if at all.

Vitamin D: Too Much May Damage Your Kidneys

Vitamin D stimulates calcium absorption in the body, and having enough is vital to health and well-being, giving the potential of preserving bones and avoiding bone illnesses like osteoporosis. Supplemental vitamin D is popular since it's difficult (if not impossible for some) to acquire enough from the diet.

Also, our bodies make vitamin D when bare skin is exposed to direct sunlight, but increased time spent indoors and widespread use of sunblock, as a necessary way to prevent skin aging and skin cancer, has minimized the amount of vitamin D many of us get from sun exposure.

Yet vitamin D pills are a complex matter. Occasionally, it might appear like rules and studies contradict one another. The reality is, excitement for vitamin D supplementation is racing the research.

For example, when healthy pre-and postmenopausal women take vitamin D (up to 400 international units, or IU), it does not always protect them from fracturing bones.

And taking large dosages is not a wise idea. In healthy adults, vitamin D blood levels greater than 100 nanograms per milliliter might stimulate excessive calcium absorption and lead to muscular discomfort, mental issues, stomach pain, and kidney stones states the Cleveland Clinic. It may also boost the risk of heart attack and stroke.

More is not always better when it comes to micronutrient supplements.

That said, vitamin D supplements may assist some people, including those at risk for deficiency such as persons who have darker skin, are living with certain health issues, and are older folks. The most recent American Geriatrics Society consensus statement specifically suggests that people older than 65 can help reduce the risk of fractures and falls by supplementing their diet with at least 1,000 IU of vitamin D per day, in addition to taking calcium supplements and eating vitamin D-rich foods.

Anyone can help bolster their vitamin D intake by spending a brief time in the sun without sunblock — about 10 to 15 minutes a day.

Keep in mind that vitamin D supplements and medications can interact with each other. Meds that don't mix well with vitamin D include the weight-loss drug orlistat (Xenical, Alli), various statins such as atorvastatin (Lipitor), thiazide diuretics (such as Hygroton, Lozol, and Microzide), and corticosteroids like prednisone (Deltasone, Rayos, Sterapred.

St. John's Wort: Avoid Drug Interactions

St. John's wort is a plant used as a tea or in capsules, with purported benefits for depression, attention-deficit hyperactivity disorder, menopause symptoms, insomnia, kidney and lung issues, obsessive-compulsive disorder, wound healing, and more.

Small studies have shown St. John's wort to be effective at treating mild depression. For example, a review of short-term studies looked at 27 clinical trials with about 3,800 patients and suggested that the herbal remedy worked as well as certain antidepressants at decreasing symptoms of mild to moderate depression.

But, The biggest issue with St. John's wort is its medication interactions. A study found that 28 percent of the time St. John's wort was prescribed between 1993 and 2010, it was administered in dangerous combinations with antidepressant or anti-anxiety medication, statins, the blood-thinning drug warfarin (Coumadin), or oral contraceptives. For example, combining St. John's wort with an antidepressant can cause serious complications, including a life-threatening increase in the brain chemical serotonin

Taking St. John's wort may also reduce the effectiveness of other medications, including birth control pills, chemotherapy, HIV or AIDS medication, and medicine to prevent organ rejection after a transplant. Before taking St. John's wort, read up on potential drug interactions, and ask your doctor about the risks and benefits of this supplement, as well as how it compares to your other options.

Calcium: The Excess May Settle in Your Arteries

Calcium is essential for a strong skeleton, but as with all nutrients, too much of this mineral may be harmful. More than 2,500 mg per day for adults ages 19 to 50, and more than 2,000 mg per day for individuals 51 and over, can lead to problems.

With calcium supplements, hardened arteries, or atherosclerosis, and a higher risk for heart disease, are risks, though research is mixed.

Get calcium from your diet if you can, noting that research shows that calcium is better absorbed through food than through supplements. In a study, researchers analyzed a group of about 5,450 healthy adults' calcium intake and screened their hearts for calcium deposits associated with atherosclerosis over 10 years. They found that people who got their calcium from food had a lower risk of atherosclerosis, while calcium supplements were associated with an increased risk of atherosclerosis.

The NIH recommends 1,000 mg of calcium a day for women ages 19 to 50 and 1,200 mg a day for women 51 and older. The recommendation for men ages 19 to 70 is 1,000 mg a day and 1,200 mg a day for men 71 and older. According to the Dietary Guidelines for Americans, there are various food sources of calcium, including plain low-fat yogurt, tofu, nonfat milk, cheese, and fortified cereal and juices.

Calcium deficiency, or hypocalcemia, may be detected by routine blood tests. If you have low calcium blood levels despite having adequate dietary intake, your doctor may prescribe a calcium supplement.

Multivitamins and multiminerals: No Alternative for a Healthy Diet

Believe that a healthy lifestyle needs not only eating good-for-you meals, exercising, and getting adequate sleep but also taking a daily multivitamin-multimineral supplement. Given that an estimated one-third of adults in the United States and one-quarter of kids take them, you may be shocked to discover that the jury's still out on whether they're useful.

One study published, which examined data from nearly 40,000 women older than 19 years who were part of the Iowa Women's Health Study, found that, on average, women who took supplements had an increased risk of dying compared with women who didn't take supplements. Multivitamins performed little or nothing to protect against common malignancies, cardiovascular disease, or mortality.

Yet, other studies have revealed the advantages of taking multivitamins. For example, research indicated that regular usage of multivitamins and mineral supplements helped avoid micronutrient deficiencies that would otherwise cause health concerns.

Generally, studies on whether multivitamins genuinely benefit health are equivocal.

For women of reproductive age, taking prenatal vitamins containing folic acid is suggested by the American College of Obstetricians and Gynecologists to help avoid birth abnormalities. Multivitamins could be given by your doctor if you have malabsorption syndrome, a disease in which the body does not adequately absorb vitamins and minerals.

In general, however a supplement can never be a replacement for a good diet.

Whereas multivitamins represent a minimal risk for medication interactions, I advises that smokers and former smokers avoid taking multivitamins containing high doses of vitamin A or beta-carotene since these nutrients may raise the risk for lung cancer when eaten as supplements.

Fish Oil Supplements: Select Fish or Flaxseed Instead

High in omega-3 fatty acids, fish oil has been suggested as a strategy to prevent heart disease and other diseases. Nevertheless accumulating data reveals that fish oil supplements have unclear advantages.

For example, research published in January 2019 in The New England Journal of Medicine reported that omega-3 supplements did nothing to lower heart attacks, strokes, or deaths from heart disease among middle-aged and older men and women without any recognized risk factors for cardiovascular disease. Previous research assessed patients at high risk for cardiovascular disease and likewise revealed no benefit.

Additionally, a subsequent review and meta-analysis of 83 randomized, controlled trials, which was published in August 2019 in the journal BMJ, indicated that omega-3s, whether in supplement or meal form, didn't lower type 2 diabetes risk among the 58,000 people enrolled.

Yet it's not all gloomy news when it comes to omega-3 supplements: A major randomized, controlled experiment published in January 2022 in BMJ reveals that fish oil supplements may give health advantages when taken with vitamin D supplements, however, in this instance the benefits weren't statistically significant. The scientists noticed that this mixture, as well as vitamin D pills alone, led to a decreased incidence of autoimmune disorders such as psoriasis and rheumatoid arthritis.

Presently, there's not enough good proof for physicians to recommend fish oil supplements to every patient, however. Apart from the varied study findings, omega-3 insufficiency is exceedingly unusual in the United States. One notable medication interaction with omega-3 supplements is Coumadin (Warfarin).

Yet, many individuals fail to eat enough omega-3s in their diet for optimum health. Omega-3s play a crucial role in the synthesis of hormones that relax arterial walls, decrease inflammation, and facilitate blood clotting.

The easiest approach to receive enough, and safe, levels of omega-3s is by consuming a range of foods that are high in them. The three primary forms of omega-3s are eicosapentaenoic acid (EPA), docosahexaenoic acid (DHA), and alpha-linolenic acid (ALA). The following are some dietary sources of EPA, DHA, and ALA omega-3s:

EPA and DHA

Fish and other seafood, particularly cold-water fatty fish, such as salmon, mackerel, tuna, herring, and sardines

DHA

Fortified foods, such as certain brands of eggs, yogurt, juices, milk, and soy beverages (may contain other forms of omega-3s, depending on the brand) (may contain other forms of omega-3s, depending on the brand)

ALA

Nuts and seeds, such as flaxseed, chia seeds, and walnuts

Plant oils, such as flaxseed oil, soybean oil, and canola oil

Kava: Overuse Can Harm Your Liver

Kava is a herb that in concentrated forms has been used to treat general anxiety disorder with some success. A study suggests that the South Pacific plant can be an effective alternative treatment to prescription medication for people diagnosed with a generalized anxiety disorder (GAD). An earlier, smaller study also showed that taking kava significantly reduced anxiety compared with a placebo in people with GAD. But taking too much kava, or taking it for too long, has been linked to serious liver damage, including hepatitis, cirrhosis, and liver failure. As a result, the FDA has warned that people, especially those with liver disease or liver problems, or those who are taking drugs that can affect the liver, should talk to their healthcare practitioner before using kava. In addition, the National Center for Complementary and Integrative Health reports that heavy consumption of kava has been associated with heart problems and eye irritation.

Several drugs may interact with kava, from anticonvulsants to anti-anxiety medications, and any drug metabolized by the liver. What's more, those taking kava ought to avoid drinking alcohol owing to probable liver injury.

Soy Isolate: Caution With Estrogen?

Tofu, tempeh, and soy milk are all healthy plant-based sources of protein, fiber, and other vital elements. Some women also consume soy in supplement form because the plant contains estrogen-like substances called isoflavones that are known to help ease symptoms of menopause. Nevertheless, some health professionals have voiced concerns that the isoflavones in soy supplements may lead to an increased risk of breast cancer.

The good news is that large-scale studies of people have not found any increased breast cancer risk from consuming entire soy foods, such as tofu and edamame, in moderation.

Indeed, research published in March 2017 in the journal Cancer looked at 6,235 breast cancer survivors and associated eating the equivalent of one serving of soybeans a week with a 21 percent decreased risk of mortality from all causes over the roughly 10-year follow-up period.

Yet not enough study has been done on soy protein isolate (SPI) the powder generated by isolating the protein from the rest of the plant to determine its actual influence on breast cancer risk. Women with a family history of breast cancer or thyroid health issues may be more prone to these consequences. But again, this is speculative and additional research is required.

In addition to supplements, SPI is commonly found in power bars, veggie burgers, and several soups, sauces, smoothies, and morning cereals.

The final line: Although current studies show that whole-food intakes of soy don't enhance breast cancer risk, the judgment is still out. Before adding any supplement to your health and wellness program, explore your choices with your healthcare team and other health specialists to weigh the possible dangers and advantages of your unique circumstances.

CHAPTER 4: VITAMINS AND YOUR DIET

It's common to resort to supplements in an effort to replenish your body with nutrients you believe may be lacking from your diet. But, going to supplements without first addressing the quality of your food may not get you far. Supplements may help cover gaps, but it's always ideal to acquire most of your vitamins and minerals via a good and balanced diet.

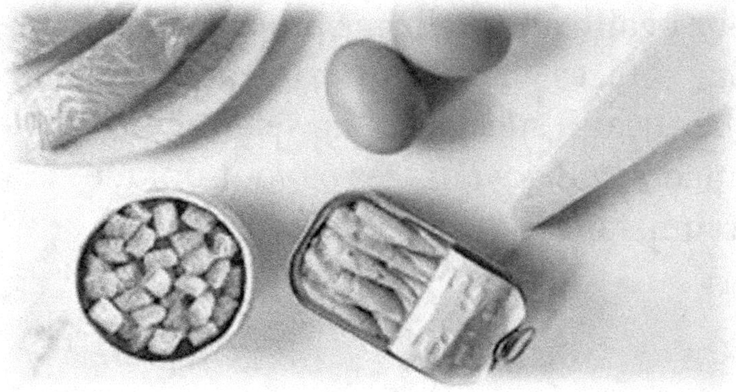

Consider adopting a food-first approach with this guide to the best dietary sources for every vitamin and mineral. You'll see that several overlaps and veggies show as a top source for practically every vitamin.

Best Multivitamins

Vitamin A

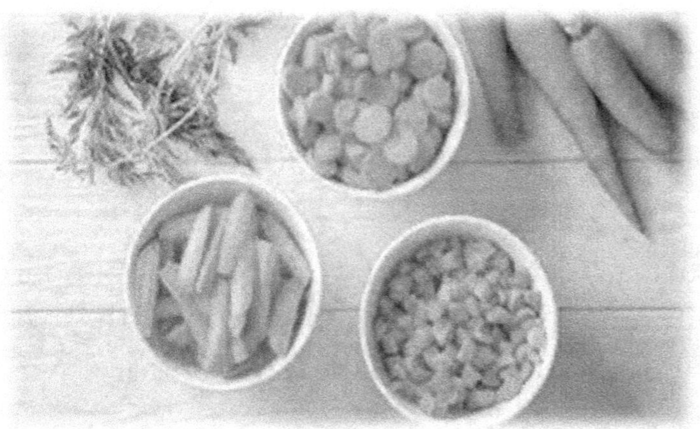

Vitamin A is a single vitamin, although two forms are present in the diet. Preformed vitamin A, which your body can utilize instantly, is present in animal diets. Provitamin A is present in plant foods, and it's a precursor to the sort of vitamin A your body can utilize. Beta-carotene is the most typical example of provitamin A.

To prevent vitamin A insufficiency in your diet, consume these foods rich in vitamin A:

- Eggs
- Meat, particularly organ meats such as liver
- Fish
- Fortified milk
- Fortified cereals

Carrots, sweet potatoes, bell peppers, cantaloupe, squash, mangos, and other red, yellow, and orange plant foods

Dark, leafy greens such as kale, spinach, arugula

Broccoli

Vitamin B

The B vitamins are a collection of eight vital nutrients people require to promote health. They're all put into one family of vitamins since they have similar qualities and are present in many of the same foods.

The eight B vitamins include:

- Vitamin B1 (thiamine)
- Vitamin B2 (riboflavin)
- Vitamin B3 (niacin)
- Vitamin B5 (pantothenic acid)
- Vitamin B6 (pyridoxine)
- Vitamin B7 (biotin)
- Vitamin B9 (folate and folic acid)
- Vitamin B12) (cyanocobalamin)

The greatest dietary sources of B vitamins are:

B1: Organ meats (such as liver and kidney), eggs, nuts, seeds, whole grains, enhanced grains, legumes, peas

B2: Eggs, dairy products, organ meats, leafy greens, lean meats, legumes, nuts

B3: Eggs, salt-water fish, poultry, fortified and whole grains, beans, avocados, potatoes

B5: Cabbage family veggies (broccoli, cabbage, brussels sprouts, kale), eggs, organ meats, poultry, milk, mushrooms, legumes, lentils, white potatoes, sweet potatoes, whole grains

B6: Beef and poultry, nuts, whole grains, avocado, bananas, legumes

B7: Chocolate, egg yolks, beans, almonds, dairy milk, organ meats, pig, yeast

B9: Asparagus, broccoli, and other cabbage-family greens, leafy greens, beets, brewer's yeast, fortified grains, lentils, oranges, wheat germ, peanuts

B12: Eggs, dairy products, chicken, beef, pig, seafood, organ meats, fortified meals (such as fortified plant pints of milk) (such as fortified plant pints of milk)

Vitamin C; sliced citrus oranges on a picnic table

Well recognized for boosting immune health, vitamin C also aids in the growth, development, and repair of many tissues in your body. Vitamin C is a key element of the structure of your skin, tendons, ligaments, and blood vessels, and it helps to produce scar tissue in reaction to traumas.

To make sure you're receiving enough vitamin C in your diet, consume lots of these vitamin C-rich foods:

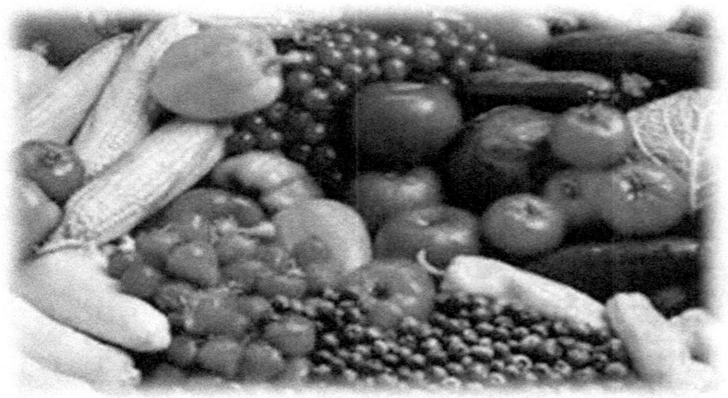

> ➢ Citrus fruits, including oranges, lemons, limes, and grapefruit

- Semi-acidic fruits, such as mangoes, papayas, kiwi, pineapple, and cantaloupe
- A variety of berries, including strawberries, blackberries, blueberries, cranberries, and raspberries
- Broccoli, brussels sprouts, cabbage, lettuce, turnip greens, spinach, collard greens, and cauliflower
- Sweet potatoes
- Winter squash varieties
- Peppers, particularly red and green variations
- Tomatoes and tomato products

Vitamin D

The absolute greatest source of vitamin D is sunlight, although lots of foods include trace levels of vitamin D to support a well-rounded diet. It's hard to obtain enough vitamin D from diet alone, so it's a good idea to be outdoors for a few minutes each day in addition to prioritizing these foods.

> - Fatty fish, such as tuna, mackerel, and salmon
> - Egg yolks
> - Beef liver
> - Mushrooms
> - Fortified milk
> - Cheese made with enriched milk
> - Additional fortified meals, such as orange juice, cereal, soy milk, and yogurt

Vitamin E

Vitamin E is an antioxidant important for numerous body activities, including the synthesis of red blood cells. Deficiency in vitamin E may lead to issues such as nerve damage, muscular weakness, loss of motor control, decreased immunological function, and eye impairments.

The top dietary sources of vitamin E are:

> - Nuts, notably peanuts, almonds, and hazelnuts

> ➢ Seeds, especially pumpkin seeds and sunflower seeds
> ➢ Some vegetable oils, including wheat germ oil, safflower oil, sunflower oil, and soybean oil
> ➢ Leafy green vegetables
> ➢ Mangos
> ➢ Avocados
> ➢ Asparagus
> ➢ Red bell pepper
> ➢ Fortified foods

Vitamin K

Vitamin K is mainly a coagulant, which means it helps blood clot. Without vitamin K, you would lose too much blood even from a little cut or scratch. Individuals on blood-thinning drugs should speak to their doctor about vitamin K before increasing their usage. If it's safe for you to consume additional vitamin K-containing foods, consider adding these sources to your diet:

> ➢ Eggs
> ➢ Poultry, pork, beef, and organ meat

> - Leafy green vegetables, such as kale, spinach, arugula, Swiss chard, lettuce, collard greens, and turnip greens
> - Broccoli, cabbage, brussels sprouts, cauliflower

Minerals

In addition to vitamins, the human body requires several minerals to function optimally. Mineral deficiencies are often responsible for symptoms like fatigue, poor sleep, low moods, and lack of focus.

You need two types of minerals to support your health: macrominerals, which you need in large amounts, and trace minerals, which you need in smaller quantities. The macrominerals include calcium, phosphorus, magnesium, sodium, potassium, chloride, and sulfur. Trace minerals include iron, manganese, copper, iodine, zinc, cobalt, fluoride, and selenium.

Calcium; close up of milk pouring into a clear glass

Calcium is the most prevalent mineral in the human body you need lots of it to maintain your bones and teeth healthy, as well as support muscle and nerve function. The best sources of calcium include:

- Dairy products
- Leafy greens
- Sardines and canned salmon, due to their edible bones
- Almonds
- Tofu cooked with calcium
- Whey protein
- Fortified foods, such as cereal or flour-based products

Phosphorus; close up shot of shrimp and oysters on a chilled platter

Second, only to calcium in terms of abundance, phosphorus makes up 1% of your body weight and is present in every cell in your body. Phosphorus helps form your bones and teeth, makes protein for tissue growth and repair, and produces the molecules your cells use for energy. These foods contain ample phosphorus:

> ➢ Beef, pig, poultry, eggs, and organ meats
> ➢ Milk, yogurt, cheese, and other dairy items
> ➢ Seafood

Many plant diets include phosphorus, but most plants store the element as phytic acid, which humans can't digest or absorb. The greatest method to acquire phosphorus is via animal meals.

Magnesium; dark chocolate baker's chocolate on a wooden countertop

Like the other macrominerals, magnesium promotes neuron and muscle function, as well as bone and heart health. You may find magnesium in:

> ➢ Whole grains
> ➢ Most fruits
> ➢ Dark chocolate
> ➢ Avocados

> Nuts, particularly almonds, Brazil nuts, and cashews
> Most seeds
> Peas and legumes
> Soy products, such as tofu and tempeh

Manganese; seared tofu in a bowl

This trace mineral is a cofactor for numerous enzymes, which means it plays a part in many chemical events that occur in your body, including the metabolism of carbohydrates and protein. The top food sources of manganese are:

> Clams, oysters, and mussels
> Brown rice and other whole grains
> Leafy greens
> Sweet potatoes
> Soybeans and soy foods, such as tofu
> Chickpeas with lima beans
> Pineapple
> Coffee and tea

Copper; whole grain bread, cereal, rice, and pasta portioned out in a white serving dish

Like manganese, copper is a cofactor for numerous enzymes. It's also crucial for appropriate brain development and connective tissue integrity. Here's where to locate copper in food:

- ➢ Whole grain goods
- ➢ Shellfish
- ➢ Chocolate
- ➢ Organ meats
- ➢ Nuts and seeds

Iodine; hand sprinkles salt into a kettle of boiling water

Your body requires iodine for effective thyroid function: Without it, your body can't generate enough thyroid hormones. Iodine is particularly vital for newborns and pregnant women since this element is critical to bone and brain growth.

The principal source of iodine in the American diet is iodized salt. If you eat a lot of salt, you probably receive enough iodine.

But in case you don't, you may obtain iodine in these additional foods:

> ➢ Fish and seafood
> ➢ Cheese, yogurt, milk, and other dairy items

Cobalt

Cobalt is present in the body as part of vitamin B-12 and helps your body metabolize and absorb the vitamin. Most meals contain minor levels of cobalt, however, diets rich in vitamin B-12 are especially high in cobalt.

Fluoride

Fluoride maintains your teeth healthy and strong. It also encourages new bone development, so it's particularly vital for newborns and youngsters. Most drinking water includes fluoride, however, if you have well water, it may not be fluoridated. In addition to water, you may acquire fluoride from:

Seafood (the ocean contains sodium fluoride)

> Coffee and tea
> Any foods prepared with fluoridated water

Selenium

Selenium protects cells from damage, promotes reproductive health and thyroid function, and supports DNA production. The most potent food source of selenium is Brazil nuts, and these can actually cause selenium toxicity if consumed too often. Other sources of food high in selenium include:

> Tuna, halibut, and sardines
> Shrimp
> Beef, pork, and chicken
> Whole grains
> Eggs
> Beans, legumes, and lentils

CHAPTER 5: VITAMINS AND YOUR LIFESTYLE

Whether you are an active daily workout enthusiast, or simply a weekend warrior, a critical aspect of attaining your physical fitness objectives and an overall healthy lifestyle is ensuring that you are fulfilling your nutritional requirements. As part of maintaining a healthy active lifestyle, a diet rich in nutrient-dense foods is vital to sustaining energy and nutritional needs. But, supplementation is frequently required to fill in the gaps and assist sustain a healthy lifestyle, particularly if daily movement is a part of your routine!

Does My Diet Have Nutritional Gaps?

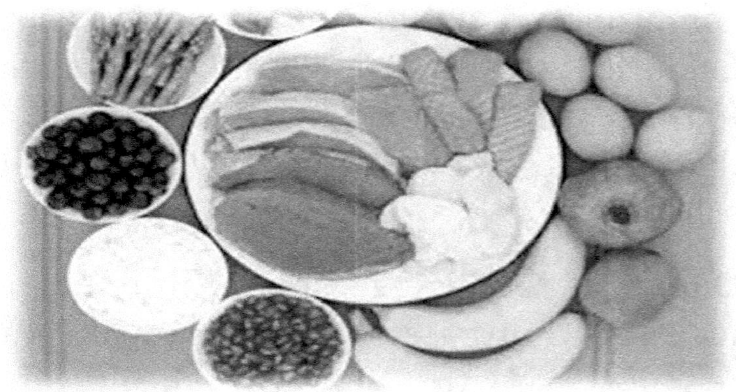

There are several elements to consider in relation to the nutritional needs of people, particularly those who lead extremely active, demanding lives. If an active individual or athlete is restricting calorie intake, following a strict weight loss program, eliminating foods or food groups from his/her diet, and/or has a low intake of key micronutrients, he/she may be at great risk for having inadequate micronutrient intake and suboptimal nutrition in their diet.

As a consequence of irregular eating habits or an imbalanced diet, regular exercise performance may be compromised. Eating a nutritious, balanced meal is an essential component for excellent health and for maintaining a demanding, but regular workout schedule.

One of our most suggested healthy living ideas is to discuss a dietary supplement regimen with your healthcare professional or Registered Dietitian/Nutritionist to explore how to best satisfy nutritional needs, maintain an active lifestyle, and promote optimum health.

Which Vitamins Promote a Healthy, Active Lifestyle?

Multivitamins

A daily multivitamin serves to assist with filling in nutrient gaps in your diet and to help satisfy the nutritional needs of active adults. To obtain the most multivitamin advantages, consider picking one depending on age and gender.

B Vitamins

A B complex supplement promotes cellular energy production. B vitamins assist transform the food you consume into energy, as well as aid promote appropriate nervous system function. Energetic individuals or athletes with greater energy demands need a balanced diet that includes a range of foods and may also consider adding a B complex vitamin to their daily supplement routine.

Antioxidants

Antioxidants help neutralize free radicals in the body to protect healthy cells from damage.

Activity may raise oxygen consumption by 10- to 15-fold, inflicting "oxidative stress" on your muscles and cells — especially during long durations of exercise.

Antioxidants act to help neutralize free radicals and typically work together in the body for the best effectiveness.† For example, vitamins C and E make a great antioxidant duo, as does vitamin C and alpha lipoic acid, to name a few. Taking a turmeric curcumin supplement is also known to provide antioxidant benefits.

Calcium & Vitamin D

Calcium and Vitamin D enhances bone health for persons with an active lifestyle. Calcium is a vital element for helping to create and strengthen healsthy bones whereas vitamin D is necessary for the correct absorption of calcium.

Calcium also has additional vital responsibilities for athletes and "weekend warriors," which include aiding with nerve transmission and muscular contraction. Excellent dietary sources of calcium include dairy products like milk, yogurt, and cheese, as well as leafy greens like kale, broccoli, mustard, and turnip greens.

Together with a balanced diet consisting of nutritious foods, supplementation with calcium and vitamin D may be recommended if dietary consumption of these minerals is inadequate, particularly in females.

Magnesium

Magnesium helps energy metabolism. Magnesium is the fourth most prevalent mineral in the body, with 50 to 60% stored in our bones, 1% detected in our blood, and the remainder of magnesium stored in cells and tissues.

Most commonly identified as an electrolyte and touted for its role in maintaining mineral balance, magnesium plays a key role in many bodily functions. Like the B vitamins, magnesium helps our systems break down the food we ingest. Magnesium is required by cells to produce ATP (adenosine triphosphate), the body's main source of energy.

Magnesium is also involved in over 300 essential metabolic functions, making this mineral a key player in cellular energy production and an essential component of good health. Despite the health benefits of magnesium, many American adults fail to consume the recommended daily amount (RDA) (RDA).

A magnesium supplement, such as Nature Made Magnesium 250 mg Liquid Softgels, may help fill nutrient gaps for this essential mineral.

A Healthy Lifestyle

A better life begins with a healthy lifestyle. Combining a healthy workout program and a nutritional diet is vital to promoting a healthier lifestyle. Take care of what you eat every day and adopt a balanced diet rich in whole foods, particularly complex carbs from vegetables, fruit, and whole grains. Lean protein and healthy fat meals are wonderful additions to a sports-friendly diet. It is also crucial to choose the proper dietary supplements to replace any vitamin shortages, maintain energy, and aid your body for each day of active life!

CHAPTER 6: THE FUTURE OF VITAMINS

Within the recent decade, methods of evidence-based medicine, with its strong emphasis on randomized controlled trials (RCT), have been extended to nutrition research and policy. Nevertheless, there are fundamental discrepancies between the data that may be gained for the testing of medications using RCTs and that required for the formulation of nutritional needs or dietary guidelines:

1) Medical interventions are designed to cure a disease not produced by their absence, while nutrients prevent dysfunction that would result from their inadequate intake;

2) Drug effects are generally intended to be large and with a limited scope of action, while nutrient effects are typically broad in scope and comparably small in effect size;

3) drug effects can be tested against a non-exposed (placebo) control group, whereas it

is impossible and/or unethical to attempt to use a zero-intake group for nutrient trials;

4) Therapeutic drugs are intended to be efficacious within a relatively short term while the impact of nutrients on the reduction of risk of chronic disease may require decades to demonstrate.

Not surprisingly, RCTs studying the impact of micronutrient supplementation on the prevention of multi-factorial chronic illnesses have most commonly failed to demonstrate meaningful benefits. Yet, there is significant epidemiological evidence relating higher micronutrient consumption (through food and/or supplements) to lowering the chances of a variety of disorders.

Such RCTs (and subsequent meta-analyses) are consequently typically problematic, not so much in their conduct as in their design. For example, the control group's consumption of the nutrient under research may not be low enough, or the participants in the treatment group may already have an adequate intake of the nutrient at the beginning of the study (thus reducing the need for supplementation).

It is also impossible to allow the nutrient under research to reveal its own right impact if the treatment group does not already have a sufficient intake of other necessary nutrients. For all these reasons, it would be good to develop some alternatives to RCTs that better represent people's eating habits and the distinctive properties of nutrients as well as acknowledge the need to cope with uncertainty coming from circumstances when we are unable to acquire data from RCTs.

We cannot be as certain in nutrition recommendations as we can in those for medications (and nutrients with a high benefit-risk ratio may need less proof of effectiveness). Unlike with medications, where unequivocal proof of effectiveness should always be needed, judgments concerning nutritional recommendations should instead be based on whether the observational data connects inadequate (or excessive) consumption to likely damage.

The insights obtained from the past 100 years of vitamin research and its uses have contributed substantially to our basic knowledge of biology and, more crucially, to the promotion of human health. There is no reason to expect that the next 100 years will be any less beneficial if we are dedicated to preparing for them, especially by shifting four essential dietary paradigms:

First, we must get beyond the premise of avoiding vitamin deficits and inadequacies. We must instead concentrate on developing health and attaining optimum physiological function. Each essential vitamin possesses different concentration thresholds for its variety of effects, and the required balance needed to achieve each has yet to be fully defined.

Second, we must apply the approaches and methods of "-omics" (e.g., metabolomics and proteomics) and systems biology research in order to define the dynamic role of vitamins and their broad array of genomic, molecular, and biochemical interactions. Such effort is important to comprehend the multitude of vitamin effects and to finally implement them directly at the level of the person.

Finally, we must reform the notion of evidence-based nutrition, moving away from its existing hierarchical structure to acknowledging in a complete and integrated fashion the contributions of each kind of approach to study. To adhere to the single gold standard of the randomized controlled trial ignores both how we have moved forward so productively over the last 100 years and the vital information that can be obtained from basic research and other human studies; further, it acts to stifle innovation in both scientific and regulatory affairs.

We must understand that changes in the supply and distribution of food during the next century are likely to be at least as dramatic as those that have occurred during this one. For example, inescapable environmental limits will necessitate that more food protein is produced from plant rather than animal sources, a move that would directly affect dietary supplies of vitamins.

In order to face the task of attaining global health by 2112 amid a population of 9 billion people, we must come up with innovative and creative methods in which individuals in academia, industry and governmental and non-governmental organizations may work together to successfully manage these four changes.

CONCLUSION

In conclusion, "Vitamins: The Missing Link in Your Health" gives an in-depth analysis of the key vitamins, their sources, functions, and health benefits. The book underlines the necessity of keeping a balanced and diverse diet to guarantee optimal consumption of important vitamins and minerals. It also covers the consequences of vitamin deficiency and the facts about vitamin supplementation.

Overall, this book is a fantastic resource for anybody trying to enhance their health and well-being. By knowing the function of vitamins in the body and how to get them via food and supplementation, readers can take control of their health and avoid the hazards of vitamin shortages.

As the title says, vitamins are the missing link in many people's health, and this book offers a complete guide to bridging that gap. With its approachable writing style and evidence-based information, "Vitamins: The

Missing Link in Your Health" is a vital read for anybody trying to enhance their health and well-being.